Contents

Acknowledgements

Many individuals and organisations contributed to this guide and provided invaluable experience and guidance. In particular, I would like to thank members of the project advisory group and all those who contributed to the pilot work.

Members of the project advisory group

Penny Banks (King's Fund); Rose Cofie (Department of Health); Andrew Cozens (Association of Directors of Social Services); Vicky Daybell (The Princess Royal Trust for Carers); Kulbir Gill (Alzheimer's Concern, Ealing); Louise Hillsley (Alzheimer's Disease Society); Adrian Lovett (North Yorkshire Health Authority); Janice Miles (NHS Confederation); Imelda Redmond (Carers UK); Peter Scott-Blackman (National Black Carers Workers Project); Pauline Shelley (Contact-A-Family); Alison Thompson (Crossroads Caring for Carers); and Stephen Wexler (The Princess Royal Trust for Carers).

Pilot work contributors

We carried out extensive pilot work in various parts of the country. These people made significant contributions to the guide, including commenting on, and testing, early versions:

Brent

Christine Cooper (Brent Triangle); Enid Jackson (Friends of Afro Caribbean Carers and Sufferers of Dementia); Sheila Karania (Asian People with Disabilities Alliance); Jane Lindo (Wembley Centre for Health and Care); Alison Linyard (Brent Carers Centre); Usha Prema (Harrow & Brent Health Authority); Meena Saleem (Asian People with Disabilities Alliance); Vernal Scott (Brent Social Services); Bob Ward (Brent Crossroads); members of the Brent Carers Priority Action Group; and the staff team, Board members and users of the Brent Carers Centre.

Ealing

Kulbir Gill and Catherine Tam (Alzheimer's Concern Ealing)

Hillingdon

Bernadette Zuiziakowska and Hardeep Jaj (Hillingdon Carers)

Good is Your
ce to Carers?

CHECKING QUALITY STANDARDS

CARER SUPPORT SERVICES

DEN

DG 02242/71

The King's Fund is an independent charitable foundation working for better health, especially in London. We carry out research, policy analysis and development activities, working on our own, in partnerships, and through grants. We are a major resource to people working in health, offering leadership and education courses; seminars and workshops; publications; information and library services; a specialist bookshop; and conference and meeting facilities.

Published by
King's Fund
11–13 Cavendish Square
London W1G 0AN
www.kingsfund.org.uk

© King's Fund 2002

Charity registration number: 207401

First published 2002

ISBN 1 85717 465 8

A CIP catalogue record for this book is available from the British Library

Available from:

King's Fund Bookshop
11–13 Cavendish Square
London W1G 0AN
Tel: 020 7307 2591
Fax: 020 7307 2801
www.kingsfundbookshop.org.uk

North West

Margaret Brewster (Carers' Partnership, Bury Metro); Joanne Brockway (Crossroads Caring for Carers, Bury); Maureen Hunter (Knowsley Carers Centre); Dilwyn James (Sefton Carers Centre); Kim Lowden (Knowsley Primary Care Groups); Maureen Mellor (St Helens Carers Project); Ged Newport (Knowsley Young Carers Project); Julie Parrish (Rochdale Social Services); Dorothy Roberts (St Helens Carers Project); Irene Sargeant (Bury Social Services); Carole Swift (St Helens Social Services); Sharon West (Trafford Social Services); Alan Wilks (Carers' Partnership, Bury Metro); Tom Wolstencroft (Rochdale Social Services & Bury & Rochdale Health Authority); and carers and staff from the North West who attended a workshop on the standards and ways of monitoring them.

Surrey

Thora Ascough (Carers' Support Mole Valley); John Bangs (Surrey Social Services); Geraldine Bolam (Action for Carers Surrey); Sarah Bowley (Action for Carers Surrey); Jane Brooks (Carers' Support Mole Valley); Jan Burden (Carers' Support Elmbridge); Wendy Cannon (Elmbridge Relief Carers Scheme); Janice Clarke (Action for Carers Surrey); Anthony Day (Carers' Support Waverley); Philip Etherton (Dorking & District Alzheimer's Society); Desiree Linnell-Cook (Carer); Bob Mitchell (Carers' Support Elmbridge); Melanie Poussicott (Elmbridge Relief Carers Scheme); Jane Thornton (Carers' Support Guildford); Roy Woolliscroft (Surrey Heath Carers); and carers and staff from Surrey who attended a workshop on the standards and ways of monitoring them.

I want to express particular appreciation to Penny Banks for her tireless support for the work, for keeping me on track, and for providing guidance and inspiration at crucial stages; Alison Linyard for supporting and co-ordinating the work in Brent; and John Bangs for supporting and co-ordinating the work in Surrey.

This work was supported by a grant from the Department of Health.

Roger Blunden
01691 648909
rblunden@onetel.net.uk

About the guide

This guide is designed to help local carer support services check how well they are meeting the quality standards developed as part of the Government's National Strategy for Carers.[1] Individuals, local groups and service organisations can use it in a variety of ways. We do not expect you to read this guide from cover to cover, but use it as a resource for checking quality.

Quality Standards for Local Carer Support Services

The standards look at what carers get from local services. They have been written by carers and people who support them. The Government has approved the standards and published them on its Carers' website.[2] The standards feature in the guidance for the Carers and Disabled Children's Act and in the guidance for the Carers' Special Grant. Those who provide and commission services should take them seriously.

There are five quality standards and a set of essential requirements. The standards relate to:

- information
- providing a break
- emotional support
- support to care and maintain the carer's own health
- having a voice.

The essential requirements should be in place for *all* carers support services. They are:

- carers are involved in the organisation
- the service works in partnership with all local agencies
- the service is clear about its principles, aims and how these will be delivered and monitored
- all staff are appropriately trained and supported.

Each section of the standards spells out that standard in general terms and then lists a number of conditions to be met. This guide is based upon the five standards and the conditions for each.

---

[1] The National Strategy for Carers can be downloaded from the Carers' website www.carers.gov.uk/pdfs/care.pdf

[2] The standards can be downloaded from the Carers' website www.carers.gov.uk/qualitystan.htm

An important theme running through the standards is a commitment to equal opportunities and to supporting carers from minority ethnic communities, as well as new or isolated carers. These are important considerations in any assessment of the quality of a service.

Services to carers

The standards apply to any services that set out to support carers. Most obviously these include specialist carer support services such as carers' centres and carer support projects. The standards also apply to any other services that include carers' support, for example, GP's surgeries, social services departments, housing and employment services.

Who the guide is for

- individual services (for example, a carers' centre or carers' support organisation) who want to check how well they are meeting the standards
- those who commission (pay for) services (for example, social services departments or primary care trusts that contract with service organisations) who want to be satisfied that the services meet acceptable standards
- carers or local groups (for example, a local carers' forum) who want to check how well the services in their area are meeting the standards
- people and groups who are setting up new services for carers, and who want to ensure that the standards are built in from the start.

What the guide *does not* do

The standards assume that services to carers already exist, or are being planned. They give a way of checking that good quality services are on offer. They are not designed to check whether there are *sufficient* services locally, or whether *all* carers' needs are met. They were designed to check how well services are doing what they set out to do.

Services should be interested in how well they meet the standards. But they may also need to monitor legal and financial and policy aspects of the way they are run. The standards do include some *essential requirements* for service organisations, but they mainly focus on what services deliver to carers. This guide is not the only way to monitor services, but it helps a service examine how well it supports its carers.

Using the guide

You can use the guide in a number of different ways.

1 As a quick self-check

Organisations can just look at the checklists and use them to discuss how well they think they are meeting the standards.

We suggest that an individual or small group take one or more of the checklists and rate the service according to their knowledge.

This sort of self-check can be useful, but it will not give a particularly thorough or accurate picture of the service. Only a limited number of people will be involved, and they may have a vested interest in seeing things in a positive light. It is based solely on what people think; there is no evidence to support their views.

A quick self-check may well be a useful starting point, but it is unlikely to be sufficient to satisfy funders or to review the service in enough detail.

2 As a 'health check' of a service organisation

You can use the guide as a more formal 'health check' on how well your organisation is meeting the standards and action that is needed to improve things. You can involve a number of people (including carers) in this work and it will give a thorough assessment of the 'health' of the service. Some funding organisations may find this a useful way of reviewing the quality of the organisations they support. Individual services should find this 'health check' a powerful means of taking stock of their achievements and deciding priorities for developing the service.

3 As a way of reviewing the quality of a local service

Carers or local groups, such as carers' forums, can use the guide to monitor how well a local service is meeting the standards.

The portfolio approach to monitoring

Most of the standards require more than simple yes/no answers. They can be met in a variety of ways. For each standard, we suggest that you compile a portfolio of evidence to show how well the standard is met. We suggest the type of evidence you could provide.

This diagram shows the approach adopted in this guide.

PROPOSED MONITORING SYSTEM

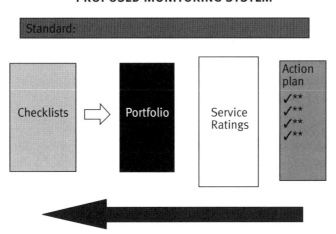

This guide contains a number of checklists to help you to assess your success in meeting aspects of the standards. We suggest information you can put into a portfolio to support your assessment.

The checklists contain simple rating scales to help you assess rate how far you meet each aspect of the standards and to highlight any priorities for action.

A simple format helps you make action plans and monitor your progress in attaining them.

Reviewing the service

We suggest that you follow these steps:

1 Familiarise yourself with the standards

Make sure that you are familiar with the standards. You can download a copy from the Government's Carers' website www.carers.gov.uk/qualitystan.htm.

2 Complete the 'Basic information' section

This section gives you space to record the overall aims of the service and something about the population you serve. It also asks how much the service reaches carers from minority ethnic populations and new or isolated carers.

3 Decide which standard(s) to review

For each standard, decide whether or not the standard applies to your organisation. For example, if your organisation only gives information to carers, the 'providing a break' standard is unlikely to apply to you. If several (or all) standards apply to your organisation, you may wish to select one or two to start with, not all five at once.

4 Do a short self-assessment

Do a short self-assessment on the selected standard(s).
An individual or small group can use the checklist as a basis for discussion. For each part of the checklist, there are five boxes to check:

- not applicable
- not met/just started
- partly met
- mostly or fully met
- action priority?

Decide which box best describes how your organisation has attained that part of the standard. The checklist includes additional guidance and definitions.

If any item on the checklist does not apply to your organisation, tick the 'Not applicable' box.

If, as you complete the checklist, you decide that any items are a priority for action, there is an additional box to check to remind you of this.

5 Collect evidence

If you are carrying out a more thorough assessment, the guide suggests evidence that you might assemble into a portfolio. Since the standards are about *carers' experience* of the support they receive, we have included some suggested *questions for carers*. You could use these as the basis of group or individual discussions, a feedback questionnaire or interviews with carers. We have suggested very basic questions, usually with a yes/no answer. We also suggest that you ask for people's comments. These comments will probably give you more useful information than the simple yes/no answers.

Action for Carers Surrey is piloting a postal questionnaire asking carers about their experience of the standards. This detailed survey could help organisations designing their own surveys. E-mail actionforcarers@talk21.com for details.

We also suggest evidence from service records and other evidence that might demonstrate your compliance with the standard. You might want to given an individual or small group the task of compiling a portfolio based on the available evidence.

If physically assembling the evidence is a major task (for example, it involves a lot of photocopying), you might simply compile a list of the evidence and where it can be found.

If you do not routinely collect feedback from carers, the *questions for carers* included in the guide suggest questions you might include in future feedback exercises.

6 Review the evidence

You can use the portfolio of evidence to assess more thoroughly how your service complies with the standards. For example, you might convene a *review group* of key stakeholders in the service to review the evidence jointly and decide how the service rates. This could include carers, service managers, service staff, trustees and service commissioners.

Reviewing the evidence can be time-consuming, particularly where you have compiled a detailed portfolio. You may find it helpful to give someone the job of summarising the information and assessing how far it complied with the standards.

Use the evidence to decide how far the service meets each of the conditions and mark this on the checklist. Tick the 'action priority' box for those areas where you want to take further action.

7 Action planning

We encourage you to use the guide to decide priorities for developing your service in line with the standards. The action planning section gives you a format for doing this.

8 Review again

Monitoring the standards is a continuing activity. You should agree how and when you will look again at your compliance with the standards. This will give you an opportunity to take stock of the progress you have made, as well as to identify further areas for development. Some services have an annual review cycle that includes feedback from carers and looks at compliance with one or more of the standards.

A REVIEW WORKSHOP

The checklists in the guide can form the basis of a workshop to review how well the standards are being met. Typically the workshop would involve carers, managers, staff, trustees, a commissioner and others with an interest in the service. A typical agenda would be:

- introductions – each person explains who they are and their interest in the service
- a brief review of the standard – use the quality standards document to outline the standard
- detailed discussion of how well each aspect of the standard is being met, using the checklists – each person can be encouraged to give their views and any supporting evidence
- priority setting and action planning – the group identifies priorities for action and decides how this will be done.

Basic information about the service

This section helps you put together basic information about your service and the population it serves. It also helps you to check how much the service complies with the *Essential requirements for quality local carer support services* set out in the National Standards.

Summary of services offered:

WHAT ARE THE OVERALL AIMS AND OBJECTIVES OF THE SERVICE?

DOES YOUR SERVICE PROVIDE THE FOLLOWING?:

☐   information

☐   a break for carers

☐   emotional support to carers

☐   support to care and maintain the carer's own health

☐   support to carers to have a voice, either individually or collectively

☐   other (summarise)

Population information

Use this space to record information about the population served by your service.

GEOGRAPHICAL AREA COVERED:

TOTAL POPULATION OF AREA (FROM CENSUS OR OTHER STATISTICS):

TOTAL NUMBER OF CARERS SUPPORTED BY YOUR ORGANISATION:

Ethnic breakdown of population (from census or other statistics)

Use whatever information you have available to compare how the ethnic mix of the general population is reflected in the carers that your organisation supports.

(The 1991 Census results should be available from local authorities. These give a breakdown of the population in terms of the following ethnic groups – White, Indian, Pakistani, Bangladeshi, Black Caribbean, Black African, Black other, Chinese, other Asian groups, Other.)

ETHNIC GROUP	% OF TOTAL POPULATION	% OF CARERS USING THE SERVICE

WHICH ETHNIC GROUPS ARE UNDER-REPRESENTED IN THE CARERS REACHED BY YOUR SERVICE?

WHAT STEPS DO YOU TAKE TO ENSURE THAT YOUR SERVICE REACHES CARERS FROM MINORITY ETHNIC POPULATIONS AND NEW OR ISOLATED CARERS?

WHAT ADDITIONAL STEPS DO YOU NEED TO TAKE TO ENSURE THAT YOUR SERVICE REACHES CARERS FROM MINORITY ETHNIC POPULATIONS AND NEW OR ISOLATED CARERS?

Essential requirements

The Quality Standards for Local Carer Support Services contain a set of four essential requirements that all services should meet. Use the space below to assess how far you meet these requirements, and tick the 'action priority' box to highlight any priority areas for action.

1 **ESSENTIAL REQUIREMENTS FOR QUALITY LOCAL CARER SUPPORT SERVICES** ***All*** carer support services need to demonstrate that they meet the essential requirements	not met/just started	partly met	mostly/fully met	action priority?
1. Carers are involved in the organisation Carers have an effective voice in service design, management, delivery, monitoring and continuous improvement	☐	☐	☐	☐
All carers have the opportunity to be involved	☐	☐	☐	☐
2. The service works in partnership with all local agencies The service is part of a joint approach to ensure carers obtain co-ordinated support and are not passed from pillar to post	☐	☐	☐	☐
3. The service is clear about its principles, aims and how these will be delivered and monitored The service has clear principles (*see notes opposite*)	☐	☐	☐	☐
The service has clearly defined aims and objectives	☐	☐	☐	☐
The service has arrangements for monitoring and evaluation which include feedback from carers	☐	☐	☐	☐
The service has a system to record any shortfall or preferences that cannot be met	☐	☐	☐	☐
The service has a complaints procedure	☐	☐	☐	☐
4. All staff are appropriately trained and supported All staff, including reception staff, volunteers and trustees are given relevant training	☐	☐	☐	☐
All staff and volunteers receive ongoing support and supervision	☐	☐	☐	☐

Notes on essential requirements

 ### Carers are involved in the organisation

Carers should have the opportunity to be involved whatever their age, gender, sexuality, disability or religion, from all local black and minority ethnic groups, unless there are very specific reasons for delivering a specialist service to one group of people, for example, a women's self help group.

 ### The service works in partnership with all agencies

These include local voluntary, statutory and private agencies.

 ### The service is clear about its principles, aims and how these will be delivered and monitored

Service principles should include:

- sensitivity to individual needs
- treating people with courtesy and respect
- recognising carers as partners
- not assuming that carers wish to be carers
- confidentiality
- promoting self determination
- not creating dependency.

The service's complaints procedure should ensure that it responds promptly to any problems and takes corrective action.

 ### All staff are appropriately trained and supported

Training should include what it is like to be a carer.

Standard 1 Information

STANDARD **1** INFORMATION	not applicable	not met/just started	partly met	mostly/fully met	action priority?
Any service providing information to carers gives information that is comprehensive, accurate and appropriate, accessible and responsive to individual needs					
a) Comprehensive [1] The service gives a wide range of information about all local services and the carer's right to an assessment OR the service offers easy signposting to other sources of expert information	☐	☐	☐	☐	☐

Notes:

[1] Carers should be able to get information on health, social, financial, legal and practical support. Information about charges should be available.

Where the service does not hold information, there should be easy signposting to other sources of expert information (for example, for people with specific conditions) and advice from trained staff.

Portfolio evidence that information is comprehensive

The following types of evidence would indicate that this aspect of the standard has been mostly or fully met:

 Feedback from carers *(ideas for questions on page 23)*

Most carers approached indicate that they can get all the information they need.

 A leaflet or brochure that describes the range of information available

There are no major gaps in available information, or if gaps are identified, it is clear how carers are signposted to other sources of expert information.

 A review of the information resource

The service:

- has reviewed its information resource within the last six months
- it can demonstrate that a comprehensive range of information is available, either directly or by signposting to other sources.

 Review of staff training and support

Records of staff training and support show that the service emphasises the importance of ensuring that carers get good quality information about services and the right to an assessment.

 Comments or complaints

There is a record of comments from carers or other professionals indicating that:

- there is general satisfaction with the range of information available
- the service has addressed any complaints or concerns about this.

STANDARD **1** INFORMATION **Any service providing information to carers gives information that is comprehensive, accurate and appropriate, accessible and responsive to individual needs**	not applicable	not met/just started	partly met	mostly/fully met	action priority?
b) Accurate and appropriate [2] Information is accurate, reliable, consistent and up-to-date	☐	☐	☐	☐	☐
Different methods of information-giving, including face-to-face discussions, are offered	☐	☐	☐	☐	☐
Notes:					

[2] It is not possible to check the accuracy of all information all the time, but the service should have some form of review in place, for example reviewing the accuracy of a sample of contact information every six months.

It will not be appropriate to offer different methods of information-giving if the service is exclusively a telephone helpline or a website.

Portfolio evidence that information is accurate and appropriate

The following types of evidence would indicate that this aspect of the standard has been mostly or fully met:

 Feedback from carers *(ideas for questions on page 23)*

Most carers approached indicate that the information they receive is accurate and up-to-date, and that they have the chance to discuss it with someone face-to-face.

 A leaflet or brochure that describes the range of information available

This makes it clear to carers that face-to-face discussions are offered.

 A review of the information resource

The service:

- has reviewed its information resource within the last six months
- can demonstrate that at least 80 per cent of the information it holds directly is up-to-date and accurate
- has a written plan to review the accuracy of its information resource (perhaps on a 'rolling' basis at least once per year)
- has an action plan to address any major inaccuracies found in the information resource.

 Review of staff training and support

Records of staff training and support show that the service emphasises the importance of ensuring that carers get accurate and appropriate information.

 Comments or complaints

There is a record of comments from carers or other professionals indicating that:

- there is general satisfaction with the accuracy of information available
- the service has addressed any complaints or concerns about this.

STANDARD 1 INFORMATION Any service providing information to carers gives information that is comprehensive, accurate and appropriate, accessible and responsive to individual needs	not applicable	not met/just started	partly met	mostly/fully met	action priority?
c) Accessible 3 The service is publicised to the whole population it serves	☐	☐	☐	☐	☐
It is clear how and when the service is available and where to go for information in an emergency or out-of-hours	☐	☐	☐	☐	☐
The service is pro-active and information is delivered to carers in their own homes and communities	☐	☐	☐	☐	☐
Information is jargon-free, easy to understand and any abbreviations are explained	☐	☐	☐	☐	☐
Information is conveyed in a variety of ways suited to carers with sight, hearing, learning or other disabilities and for carers for whom English is not their first language	☐	☐	☐	☐	☐
The service can arrange access to trained interpreters and signers	☐	☐	☐	☐	☐
Carers can view their personal records and the service complies with Data Protection legislation	☐	☐	☐	☐	☐

Notes:

3 The service should try to reach people who have never associated themselves with the title of carer. Information may be sent to carers in their own homes and communities using the internet, post or phone.

For statutory services, access to carers' own records should be within the limits of Clients Access to Records legislation.

The service should review its compliance with Data Protection legislation.

Portfolio evidence that information is accessible

The following types of evidence would indicate that this aspect of the standard has been mostly or fully met:

 Feedback from carers *(ideas for questions on page 23)*

Most carers approached indicate that the information they receive is clear and available in a language they can understand.

 A leaflet or brochure that describes the range of information available

This publication:

- makes clear to carers how information is available in other languages and accessible formats (for example, through trained interpreters or signers)
- describes the availability of the service and where to go in an emergency or out-of-hours
- makes clear that carers' personal records are, where possible, written with them and accessible to them (within the limits of legislation).

A review of the information resource

This would include:

- written evidence that the information resource has been publicised to the whole population
- evidence from service records that carers from a range of communities (including minority communities) have accessed the service
- written evidence that the service has reviewed its compliance with Data Protection legislation.

Comments or complaints

There is a record of comments from carers or other professionals indicating that:

- there is general satisfaction with the accessibility of information available
- the service has addressed any complaints or concerns about this.

STANDARD **1** INFORMATION **Any service providing information to carers gives information that is comprehensive, accurate and appropriate, accessible and responsive to individual needs**	not applicable	not met/just started	partly met	mostly/fully met	action priority?
d) Responsive 4 Carers help to develop, evaluate and update the information that the service provides	☐	☐	☐	☐	☐
Carers' enquiries are answered promptly and courteously and answering services are only used as a last resort. The service sets and publishes a standard for response times	☐	☐	☐	☐	☐

Notes:

4 Enquiries from carers may be by telephone, minicom, letter, fax, e-mail or by personal visit.

Portfolio evidence that information is responsive

The following types of evidence would indicate that this aspect of the standard has been mostly or fully met:

 Feedback from carers *(ideas for questions below)*

Most carers approached indicate that the service has treated them courteously and promptly.

 A published response policy

The service publishes a response policy emphasising courtesy of response and including high standards for response times (for example, a response to all enquiries within two working days).

 A review of the information resource

Written evidence that carers are fully involved in the development of the information resource.

 Comments or complaints

There is a record of comments from carers or other professionals indicating that:

- there is general satisfaction with the responsiveness of information available
- the service has addressed any complaints or concerns about this.

FEEDBACK FROM CARERS, STANDARD 1

You should have some way of collecting feedback from a representative sample of carers (*see* Collect evidence *on page 9*).

For Standard 1, questionnaires or interviews might focus on the following questions:

- Has this service given you information about what support you can get? (Yes/No/Comments)
- Did you get all the information you needed? (Yes/No/Comments)
- Did you get the chance to discuss the information with someone face-to-face? (Yes/No/Comments)
- How clear was the information? (Could you understand it? Was it available in your language?) (Very clear/Fairly clear/Not very clear/Unclear/Comments)
- Was the information up-to-date? (Yes/No/Comments)
- Has the service dealt with your enquiries promptly? (Yes/No/Comments)
- Has the service treated you courteously? (Yes/No/Comments)
- Do you have any other comments on the information service you receive?

STANDARD 2 PROVIDING A BREAK **Any service offering a break to carers [1] works in partnership with the carer and person being supported, is flexible and gives confidence and can be trusted**	not applicable	not met/just started	partly met	mostly/fully met	action priority?
a) Works in partnership The service respects the carer and the caring relationship	☐	☐	☐	☐	☐
The service has an agreed process for dealing with any conflict between the carer and person being supported	☐	☐	☐	☐	☐
Full information is provided about the service and there are opportunities to meet staff or visit the service before the carer and person being supported make any decisions	☐	☐	☐	☐	☐
The service encourages both the carer and the person being supported to give feedback	☐	☐	☐	☐	☐

Notes:

[1] These services may be provided at home, in day or residential facilities, in community, leisure or holiday settings, or in other people's homes and include services which provide opportunities for the carer and person being supported to go away together. These are services which provide a real break and 'time off' for the carer, not an emergency response when there is a crisis.

Portfolio evidence of working in partnership

The following types of evidence would indicate that this aspect of the standard has been mostly or fully met:

 Feedback from carers *(ideas for questions on page 27)*

The service can demonstrate that it actively encourages feedback from the carer and person being supported (for example, comment cards, feedback forms).

Most carers approached indicate that the service works in partnership with them and that they are fully consulted.

 A leaflet or brochure that describes the service

This gives full information about the service and emphasises how the service works in partnership with carers.

 Policies and procedures

The service can show that it has written policies that stress how the service operates flexibly to meet carers' needs, including cultural and religious needs.

 Examples

The service can give examples of how it has operated at times to suit carers, including night time, over public holidays, mid-week starts and other non-standard length breaks.

 Comments or complaints

There is a record of comments from carers or other professionals indicating that:

- there is general satisfaction with the working relationship
- the service has addressed any complaints or concerns about this.

STANDARD **2** PROVIDING A BREAK	not applicable	not met/just started	partly met	mostly/fully met	action priority?
Any service offering a break to carers works in partnership with the carer and person being supported, is flexible and gives confidence and can be trusted					
b) Flexible and adaptable to carers' needs [2] The service is suited to the assessed needs and wishes of the carer [3]	☐	☐	☐	☐	☐
The service is flexible and can time services to suit the carer [4]	☐	☐	☐	☐	☐

Notes:

[2] Services should be flexible and adaptable in meeting the cultural needs of local carers.

[3] The assessed needs and wishes of the carer should include their cultural and religious needs.

[4] Wherever possible the service should operate at night, over public holidays, offer mid-week starts and non-standard length breaks. At a minimum the service should make every attempt to negotiate the best possible arrangements with the carer.

Portfolio evidence of flexibility

The following types of evidence would indicate that this aspect of the standard has been mostly or fully met:

 Feedback from carers *(ideas for questions below)*

Most carers approached indicate that the service is flexible enough to meet their needs.

 Policies and procedures

Policies and procedures on the allocation of support to individuals stress the flexibility of the service.

 Examples

The service can give examples of how it has provided flexible services.

 Comments or complaints

There is a record of comments from carers or other professionals indicating that:

- there is general satisfaction with the flexibility of the service
- the service has addressed any complaints or concerns about this.

FEEDBACK FROM CARERS, STANDARD 2

You should have some way of collecting feedback from a representative sample of carers. (*see* Collect evidence *on page 9*).

For Standard 2, questionnaires or interviews might focus on the following questions:

- Does this service work in partnership with you and the person you care for? Are you fully consulted about caring arrangements? (Yes/No/Comments)
- Did you get full information and a chance to meet staff or visit the service before making any decision? (Yes/No/Comments)
- Is the service flexible enough to meet your needs? (Yes/No/Comments)
- Does the service give you peace of mind? (Yes/No/Comments)
- Does the service ensure that the person you care for has interesting things to do and foster his or her independence? (Yes/No/Comments)
- Does the service treat you and the person you care for with dignity and respect? Is privacy maintained? (Yes/No/Comments)
- Do you get consistent care from one break to the next (for example, is the same care worker involved)? (Yes/No/Comments)
- Does the service meet the person's personal preferences about the way care is provided? (Yes/No/Comments)
- Does the service properly look after clothes and personal possessions? (Yes/No/Comments)

STANDARD 2 PROVIDING A BREAK **Any service offering a break to carers works in partnership with the carer and person being supported, is flexible and gives confidence and can be trusted**	not applicable	not met/just started	partly met	mostly/fully met	action priority?
c) The service gives confidence and can be trusted 5 Carers say that they get peace of mind from the service	☐	☐	☐	☐	☐
The service is sensitive to the needs and choices of the person being supported	☐	☐	☐	☐	☐
The service provides a stimulating environment that fosters independence and well being	☐	☐	☐	☐	☐
The service provides personalised care in a friendly, welcoming atmosphere	☐	☐	☐	☐	☐
The service ensures the quality of care is consistent from one break to the next	☐	☐	☐	☐	☐
The service meets the person's preferences in the way personal care is provided	☐	☐	☐	☐	☐
The service properly looks after clothes and personal possessions	☐	☐	☐	☐	☐
The service ensures that workers are appropriately trained and supervised, with relevant security checks	☐	☐	☐	☐	☐
Notes:					

5 The needs and choices of the person being supported should include their age, gender, sexuality, disability, religion, ethnicity, and personal needs and choices.

The environment should be stimulating, not simply safe, whether it is in a residential home, day service or offered through one-to-one care in someone's own home.

The service should ensure that individuals are treated with dignity and respect and that privacy is maintained.

Wherever possible the service should provide the same paid care worker or at least someone previously known to the carer and person cared for.

The person's preferences should be met in ways that do not conflict with the need to safeguard the health and safety of the person delivering the care.

Training, supervision and security checks should apply to all staff, paid or voluntary, and whether going into people's homes, residential care or day facilities.

Workers should have an understanding of what it is like to be a carer.

Portfolio evidence of carer confidence

The following types of evidence would indicate that this aspect of the standard has been mostly or fully met:

 Feedback from carers *(ideas for questions on page 27)*

Most carers approached report that the service:

- gives them peace of mind
- stimulates the person supported and promotes their independence
- treats the carer and person cared for with respect and dignity
- respects confidentiality
- provides consistent care
- meets personal preferences
- properly looks after clothes and personal possessions.

 Policies and procedures

Written policies and procedures, including staff training, aimed at promoting the items in the above checklist.

 Examples

Examples of how the service has supported individuals in a way that has consistently promoted independence, dignity and respect.

 Records

Staff training records showing that the items in the above checklist have been attended to. Documentary evidence that relevant security checks have been done.

 Comments or complaints

There is a record of comments from carers or other professionals indicating that:

- there is general satisfaction with service
- the service has addressed any complaints or concerns about this.

Standard 3 | Emotional support

STANDARD **3** EMOTIONAL SUPPORT [1] **Any service offering emotional support to carers, either on a one-to-one basis or in a group, is sensitive to individual needs, confidential, offers continuity and is accessible to all carers**	not applicable	not met/just started	partly met	mostly/fully met	action priority?
a) Sensitive to individual needs The service offers a safe and non-judgemental environment for carers to share feelings, confidences, information and knowledge [2]	☐	☐	☐	☐	☐
If carers have said that they want to run their own support groups, this is supported	☐	☐	☐	☐	☐
Any service described as a counselling service [3] is delivered by suitably qualified and supported professionals [4]	☐	☐	☐	☐	☐
Any service offering counselling is competent to address the carers' culture, religion, preferred language, age, gender, sexuality and disability	☐	☐	☐	☐	☐
b) Confidential The service is confidential and has a code of practice [5] to ensure no breach of confidentiality	☐	☐	☐	☐	☐
Notes:					

[1] These services may include: befriending; help lines or phone contacts which offer a 'listening ear', counselling; support groups; social activities; one-to-one links with other carers; internet links.

[2] Opportunities to talk can be provided either in a group or on a one-to-one basis.

[3] Carers' services may not themselves offer counselling, but may refer people to other agencies which provide counselling.

[4] Counselling professionals are supported or accredited by a recognised professional body, such as the British Association of Counselling, or approved as culturally competent by therapists within black and minority ethnic communities.

[5] The code of practice should include agreed protocols for disclosure in relation to abuse and matters of public safety.

Portfolio evidence of emotional support

The following types of evidence would indicate that these aspects of the standard has been mostly or fully met:

 Feedback from carers *(ideas for questions on page 35)*

Most carers approached indicate that the service gives them a chance to talk things over in a safe and confidential way.

Carers state that they are happy with the way support groups are run.

Carers state that they have been supported to take over or run a group where they have wanted to do this.

Carers state that any counselling service offered meets their cultural, language and other preferences.

 A leaflet or brochure that describes the service

This gives full information about the emotional support offered and emphasises the confidentiality of the service.

 Policies and procedures

If counselling is offered, the service has a clear policy about appointing properly accredited and supported professionals, or those approved as culturally competent by therapists within black and minority ethnic communities.

There is a code of practice about confidentiality and the circumstances where information may be disclosed.

 Comments or complaints

There is a record of comments from carers or other professionals indicating that:

■ there is general satisfaction with the emotional support provided
■ the service has addressed any complaints or concerns about this.

STANDARD **3** EMOTIONAL SUPPORT **Any service offering emotional support to carers, either on a one-to-one basis or in a group, is sensitive to individual needs, confidential, offers continuity and is accessible to all carers**	not applicable	not met/just started	partly met	mostly/fully met	action priority?
c) Offers continuity The service continues to offer support when and after the person being cared for dies	☐	☐	☐	☐	☐
The service continues to offer support if needed when caring responsibilities change (for example, if the person cared for goes to live elsewhere)	☐	☐	☐	☐	☐

Notes:

Portfolio evidence of continuity

The following types of evidence would indicate that this aspect of the standard has been mostly or fully met:

 Policies and procedures

The service has a written policy about supporting carers after the person they are caring for dies or if caring responsibilities change (even if this is for a limited time period).

 Examples

Examples of how the service has supported individual carers after the person being cared for has died or when caring responsibilities have changed.

 Comments or complaints

There is a record of comments from carers or other professionals indicating:

- general satisfaction with the continuity of the service after the person being cared for has died or caring responsibilities have changed
- that any complaints or concerns have been addressed.

STANDARD **3** EMOTIONAL SUPPORT	not applicable	not met/just started	partly met	mostly/fully met	action priority?
Any service offering emotional support to carers, either on a one-to-one basis or in a group, is sensitive to individual needs, confidential, offers continuity and is accessible to all carers					
d) Accessible to all carers The service or support group is well publicised, especially to new or isolated carers	☐	☐	☐	☐	☐
Venues and times of the group are planned with local carers	☐	☐	☐	☐	☐

Notes:

Portfolio evidence of accessibility

The following types of evidence would indicate that this aspect of the standard has been mostly or fully met:

 Service records

The service can demonstrate through its records that it provides emotional support to a broad cross-section of carers, including carers from minority communities.

 Examples

There are examples of new or isolated carers receiving emotional support from the service.

The service can demonstrate how it has reached out to new or isolated carers (for example, through other services or by widely-circulated publicity material).

FEEDBACK FROM CARERS, STANDARD 3

You should have some way of collecting feedback from a representative sample of carers (*see* Collect evidence *on page 9*).

For Standard 3, questionnaires or interviews might focus on the following questions:

- Does this service give you a chance to talk over things in a safe and confidential way (for example, in a group or with a counsellor)? (Yes/No/Comments)
- If you don't get a chance to talk things over in a group or with a counsellor, is this something you would like? (Yes/No/Comments)
- Is there a support group run by carers? (Yes/No/Comments)
- Have you had the opportunity to have a support group run by carers? (Yes/No/Comments)
- Do you get counselling from the service? (Yes/No/Comments)
- Are you happy with the confidentiality of the support service? (Yes/No/Comments)
- In general, how satisfied are you with the emotional support you get from this service? (Very satisfied/Fairly satisfied/Not very satisfied/Dissatisfied/Comments)

Standard 4 | Support to care and maintain carer's own health

STANDARD 4 SUPPORT TO CARE AND MAINTAIN CARER'S OWN HEALTH **Any service that supports carers to care and to maintain their own health and well-being by offering training, health promotion and personal development opportunities and is responsive to individual needs**	not applicable	not met/just started	partly met	mostly/fully met	action priority?
The service gives up-to-date and comprehensive information about local training, [1] health and personal development opportunities [2]	☐	☐	☐	☐	☐
The service offers carers a range of opportunities for training, health and personal development, taking local culture and religion into account	☐	☐	☐	☐	☐
The service works in partnership with other local agencies to promote good health for carers [3] and to ensure that carers have appropriate training or guidance to care [4]	☐	☐	☐	☐	☐
The service works with GPs and Primary Care Teams to promote the checklist in the National Strategy for Carers (see notes opposite)	☐	☐	☐	☐	☐
The service works in partnership with other agencies to ensure that carers are supported to take up training and development opportunities (for example, by ensuring that alternative care is available)	☐	☐	☐	☐	☐
The service promotes the health needs of carers following bereavement	☐	☐	☐	☐	☐
Notes:					

[1] Training opportunities may be offered at home by health or other professionals who provide the necessary information and expertise, or through courses for carers, professionals or the public. These one-to-one sessions or courses may cover physical and mental illnesses, practical tips on caring, use of equipment, self-assertiveness, emergency and first aid.

[2] Personal development opportunities may include employment, education or social activities.

[3] Health promotion may include sessions to assist carers look after their own physical and emotional health, relaxation and other therapies.

[4] The service encourages the provision of training, health and personal development opportunities which suit the needs of local carers in content, time and delivery and take into account culture, religion, age, disability, gender and sexuality.

CHECKLIST FOR GPS AND PRIMARY CARE TEAMS

The checklist in the National Strategy for Carers asks:

- Have you identified those of your patients who are carers, and patients who have a carer?
- Do you check carers' physical and emotional health whenever a suitable opportunity arises, and at least once a year?
- Do you routinely tell carers that they can ask social services for an assessment of their own needs?
- Do you always ask patients who have carers whether they are happy for health information about them to be told to their carer?
- Do you know whether there is a carers' support group or carers' centre in your area, and do you tell carers about them?

Portfolio evidence of support

The following types of evidence would indicate that these aspects of the standard has been mostly or fully met:

 Feedback from carers *(see ideas for questions on page 39)*

Most carers approached indicate that the service has given them information about ways of looking after their own health and well-being.

Carers have taken up training and other development opportunities and found these helpful.

Carers state that they received the help and support they needed to take up training and development opportunities.

 Policies and procedures

Policy/procedures on how the service promotes the health needs of carers.

 A leaflet or brochure

This includes up-to-date information about training and development opportunities for carers.

 Service records

Numbers of carers who have been supported to take up training or development opportunities.

✓ Examples

Examples of partnership work with other agencies to promote carers' health and well-being.

Correspondence or meeting notes showing how the service has worked with GPs and Primary Care Teams to promote the checklist in the National Strategy for Carers.

Evidence of GPs and Primary Care Teams putting the checklist into practice, for example, by setting up systems to identify carers.

Examples of local arrangements to support carers attending training and development opportunities.

Examples (suitably anonymised) of the service promoting carers' health needs following bereavement.

✓ Comments or complaints

There is a record of comments from carers or other professionals indicating that:

- there is general satisfaction with the support offered to carers for their own well-being
- the service has addressed any complaints or concerns about this.

FEEDBACK FROM CARERS, STANDARD 4

You should have some way of collecting feedback from a representative sample of carers (*see* Collect evidence *on page 9*).

For Standard 4, questionnaires or interviews might focus on the following questions:

- Has the service given you information about ways you can learn more about how to look after your own health and well-being (for example, training courses)? (Yes/No/Comments)
- Have you taken up any of these opportunities (for example, been on a course)? (Yes/No/Comments)
- How relevant is the local training/guidance to your own needs? (Very relevant/Fairly relevant/Not very relevant/Not relevant at all/Comments)
- Do you get the help and support you need (for example, someone to provide care, help with transport) to get to planning meetings and training courses? (Yes/No/Comments)

Standard 5 | Having a voice

STANDARD 5 HAVING A VOICE	not applicable	not met/just started	partly met	mostly/fully met	action priority?
Any service that supports carers to have a voice as an individual and/or collectively, is accessible to all carers and can act in an independent way					
a) Supporting hidden carers [1] The service is pro-active in involving people who do not identify themselves as carers and carers from excluded communities [2]	☐	☐	☐	☐	☐

Notes:

[1] Any service supporting carers to have a voice and an ongoing dialogue with other local services needs to be pro-active to ensure hidden carers who do not identify themselves as carers and carers from excluded communities are involved. This would include, for example, carers in rural areas, black and minority ethnic carers, people with communication problems, travellers, refugees and asylum seekers.
[2] Services should actively ensure the participation of carers from all communities, whatever their age, gender, sexuality, disability or ethnicity.

Portfolio evidence of support for hidden carers

The following types of evidence would indicate that this aspect of the standard has been mostly or fully met:

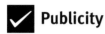 **Publicity**

Publicity material is widely available and is accessible to people from different communities.

The service can demonstrate that it has made specific efforts to reach hidden carers (for example, through local publicity, co-operation with other agencies).

 Policies and procedures

The service has an explicit policy of seeking to reach hidden carers and people from excluded communities.

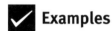 **Examples**

The service can give examples of how it has successfully reached hidden carers and people from excluded communities – for example, through posters, leaflet campaigns, outreach workers, talks to local groups, radio/TV broadcasts, other publicity campaigns.

STANDARD 5 HAVING A VOICE **Any service that supports carers to have a voice as an individual and/or collectively, is accessible to all carers and can act in an independent way**	not applicable	not met/just started	partly met	mostly/fully met	action priority?
b) Supporting carers to have a voice [3] The service provides independent one-to-one advocacy	☐	☐	☐	☐	☐
The service goes beyond the provision of information and ensures that carers can make informed choices and advocate for themselves where appropriate	☐	☐	☐	☐	☐
Staff or volunteers providing advocacy are supported, trained and accountable	☐	☐	☐	☐	☐
Advocates are suited to the individual needs, culture and ethnicity of the carer who, wherever possible, has some choice in his/her advocate	☐	☐	☐	☐	☐

Notes:

[3] An advocate is someone (paid staff member or volunteer) who is specifically trained and supported to speak on behalf of a carer, or to support him or her to speak up for themselves.

Portfolio evidence of support for individual voice

The following types of evidence would indicate that this aspect of the standard has been mostly or fully met:

 Feedback from carers *(ideas for questions on page 46)*

Most carers approached indicate that the service supports them to speak up about what is important to them as a carer.

Most carers say that they are satisfied with these support arrangements.

 Policies and procedures

Policies and procedures on the provision of advocacy include arrangements for the training and support of advocates.

 Service records

Training records for advocates show that they have been appropriately trained.

Support/supervision records for advocates show that they have been appropriately supported.

Staff records show that advocates match the cultural and ethnic backgrounds of local populations.

 Examples

The service can give examples of how individuals have been supported to speak up about their requirements and concerns.

 Comments or complaints

There is a record of comments from carers or other professionals indicating that:

- there is general satisfaction with the way individual carers have been supported to have a voice
- the service has addressed any complaints or concerns about this.

STANDARD **5** HAVING A VOICE Any service that supports carers to have a voice as an individual and/or collectively, is accessible to all carers and can act in an independent way	not applicable	not met/just started	partly met	mostly/fully met	action priority?
c) Supporting carers to have a collective voice The service involves carers from all communities and undertakes outreach work to ensure their participation	☐	☐	☐	☐	☐
The service supports carers to be involved in policy development, planning activities, service evaluation and the training of professionals. This includes providing them with accessible information about these activities	☐	☐	☐	☐	☐
The service works with other agencies to ensure that carers get emotional and practical support to take part in planning and training	☐	☐	☐	☐	☐
The service promotes independent monitoring of statutory services by carers	☐	☐	☐	☐	☐
The service actively seeks feedback from carers and passes this on to all interested and relevant parties	☐	☐	☐	☐	☐
Carers' representatives have contact with other carers to hear their views and to report progress, share ideas and gain support	☐	☐	☐	☐	☐
Carers are kept informed of the results of their involvement with services and are given reasons if their recommendations cannot be implemented	☐	☐	☐	☐	☐

Notes:

Portfolio evidence of support for collective voice

The following types of evidence would indicate that this aspect of the standard has been mostly or fully met:

 Feedback from carers *(ideas for questions on page 46)*

Most carers approached indicate that they are satisfied with the way the service supports them to take part in meetings, planning sessions, and training.

 Examples

Examples of ways in which carers have been supported to be involved in policy development, planning activities, service evaluation, or the training of professionals. These should be supported by written reports and include any information about the impact of carer involvement in these activities.

Examples of how the service has worked with other agencies to ensure that carers get support to take part in these activities.

Examples of how carers have been kept informed of the results of their involvement with services.

 Comments or complaints

There is a record of comments from carers or other professionals indicating that:

- there is general satisfaction with the way that carers have been supported to have a collective voice
- the service has addressed any complaints or concerns about this.

FEEDBACK FROM CARERS, STANDARD 5

You should have some way of collecting feedback from a representative sample of carers (*see* Collect evidence *on page 9*).

For Standard 4, questionnaires or interviews might focus on the following questions:

- Does the service help you to speak up about what is important for you as a carer? (Yes/No/Comments)
- Are you part of a group of carers who have a say about services? (Yes/No/Comments)
- How satisfied are you with the arrangements to help you speak up, either as an individual or in a group? (Very satisfied/Fairly satisfied/Not very satisfied/Dissatisfied/Comments)
- Do you get any help or support to take part in meetings, planning sessions and training (for example, help with transport, someone to look after the person you care for)? (Yes/No/Comments)
- Do you get information about planning meetings and training in a form you can understand? (Yes/No/Comments)
- Have you ever been involved in monitoring the way health or social services support carers? (Yes/No/Comments)
- Do you think services listen to what you have to say and take notice? (Yes/No/Comments)
- Do services tell you how they will respond to feedback from carers? (Yes/No/Comments)
- Do you have the chance to meet carers from other places to hear their views and share ideas? (Yes/No/Comments)

Action guidance

Use the checklists to identify priority areas for change. The following format will help ensure that good intentions for change are actually put into practice. The basis of sound action planning is:

Set clear targets – write as plainly as possible what needs to be achieved. Describe each target so that you will know when you have achieved it. For example: 'Complete a survey of carers' views on the peace of mind they get from our service' is clearer than 'Find out what carers think'.

Set a target date – agree a date when the target will be achieved.

Identify who will be responsible for ensuring that the target is met – this will not necessarily be the person who carries out all the work, just the person with responsibility to ensure that it happens.

List any resource implications – identify any budget or time implications for carrying out the work.

Agree a review date – decide when you will review progress.

A suggested format for recording your action plans is given overleaf.

An example of a completed action planning template is show below.

Standard	Condition	Target	Target date	Person responsible	Resource implications	Review date
1	Accessible	Circulate to all carers a statement of the service hours and out-of-hours and emergency contacts. Also post this on website	End March	Hilary (information co-ordinator)	One day of Hilary's time, admin support, printing, postage	3 April team meeting
3	Confidential	Draw up a confidentiality statement for approval by management group	End January	Claire (service manager)	Half a day of Claire's time. Management group time	2 Feb Mgt Group meeting

Action planning template

Standard	Condition	Target	Target date	Person responsible	Resource implications	Review date

Sources of guidance for implementing the quality standards

There are a range of sources of guidance that will be of help in putting the quality standards into practice. Some of these are listed below.

Parent organisations

Services that are part of a parent organisation (for example, the Alzheimer's Disease Society, Contact-a-Family, Crossroads Caring for Carers, Princess Royal Trust for Carers) will be able to obtain guidance and support from their organisation.

The parent organisations mentioned above were part of the project to develop this guide and are committed to putting it into practice within their services:

Alzheimer's Disease Society
Gordon House
10 Greencoat Place
London
SW1P 4ND
Tel: 020 7306 0606
Fax: 020 7306 0808
Helpline: 0845 300 0336

Contact-A-Family
209–211 City Road
London
EC1V 1JN
Tel: 020 7608 8700
Fax: 020 7608 8701
Minicom: 020 7608 8702
Helpline: 0808 808 3555 Freephone for parents and families (10am–4pm, Mon–Fri)
E-mail: info@cafamily.org.uk
Website: www.cafamily.org.uk

Crossroads Caring for Carers
10 Regent Place
Rugby
Warwickshire
CV21 2PN
Tel: 01788 573653
Fax: 01788 565498
E-mail: association.office@crossroads.org.uk
Website: www.crossroads.org.uk

The Princess Royal Trust for Carers
142 Minories
London
EC3N 1LS
Website: www.carers.org.uk

London Office
142 Minories
London
EC3N 1LB
Tel: 020 7480 7788
Fax: 020 7481 4729
E-mail: info@carers.org.uk

Glasgow Office
Campbell House
215 West Campbell Street
Glasgow
G2 4TT
Tel: 0141 221 5066
Fax: 0141 221 4623
E-mail: infoscotland@carers.org.uk

Northern Office
Suite 4, Oak House
High Street
Chorley
PR7 1DW
Tel: 01257 234 070
Fax: 01257 234 105
E-mail: infochorley@carers.org.uk

Other organisations

Carers UK

Carers UK focuses on policy advice and information about carers' issues. It has a regularly updated website and provides policy briefings, benefits advice, and information and research. It also provides a broad range of high-quality training on benefits and community care legislation to people who work with carers. Associate members receive regular briefings.

Carers UK
Ruth Pitter House
20–25 Glasshouse Yard
London
EC1A 4JS
Website: www.carersonline.org.uk
Training information, tel: 020 7566 7632
Associate Membership information, tel: 020 7490 8818

Commission for Racial Equality (CRE)

The CRE provides advice and guidance on ways of ensuring that organisations comply with race relations legislation. The CRE works with the National Council for Voluntary Organisations to run a series of free seminars for voluntary organisations to explain the implications of the new race relations legislation on the voluntary sector. The CRE has produced a draft statutory code of practice to help authorities in England and Wales meet their duty; draft good practice guides for public authorities, schools, and institutions of further and higher education; and a draft guide to ethnic monitoring for public authorities. A separate code is being prepared for authorities in Scotland.

Commission for Racial Equality
Elliot House
10–12 Allington Street
London
SW1E 5EH
Tel: 0207 828 7022
Fax: 0207 630 7605
E-mail info@cre.gov.uk
Website: www.cre.gov.uk

Croner

Croner provides a range of products that give guidance relating to legal, employment, management and other aspects of running organisations. It also provides a pack, *Management of Voluntary Organisations*, which provides guidance and advice for those involved in setting up new voluntary organisations or managing existing ones.

Croner CCH Group Limited
145 London Road
Kingston upon Thames
Surrey
KT2 6SR
Tel: 020 8547 3333
Fax: 020 8547 2638
E-mail: info@croner.cch.co.uk
Website: www.croner.cch.co.uk

Department of Health

The Department of Health supported the work on the National Standards for Carers Support Services, and the work on this guide.

Website: www.carers.gov.uk

Directory for Social Change

The Directory for Social Change helps voluntary and community organisations to thrive, by giving advice on:

- how to raise the money they need
- how to manage their resources to maximum effect
- how to influence the right people
- what their rights and responsibilities are
- how to plan and develop for the future.

The Directory has a range of publications and offers training.

Directory for Social Change
24 Stephenson Way
London
NW1 2DP
Tel: 020 7391 4900
E-mail: promo@dsc.org.uk
Website: www.dsc.org.uk

The King's Fund

The King's Fund has produced a wide range of materials relating to support for carers. It also has a comprehensive library, including books and journals relating to the management of care organisations.

The King's Fund
11–13 Cavendish Square
London
W1G 0AN
Tel: 020 7307 2400
Fax: 020 7307 2801
Website: www.kingsfund.org.uk

National Black Carer Worker Network (NBCWN)

The NBCWN has produced a *Good Practice Guide* to ensure that services meet the needs of black carers, as set out in the *Black Carers Manifesto 2000*.

Further information from:
Peter Scott-Blackman
c/o The Afiya Trust
Unit 11
27–29 Vauxhall Grove
London
SW8 1SY
Tel: 020 7582 0400

or

Elaine Powell
c/o CARES
The Carers Centre
2 Bearwood Road
Smethwick
West Midlands
B66 4HH
Tel: 0121 558 7003
E-mail: nbcwn@lycos.co.uk

National Council for Voluntary Organisations (NCVO)

The National Council for Voluntary Organisations (NCVO) is the umbrella body for the voluntary sector in England, with sister councils in Wales (Wales Council for Voluntary Action, WCVA), Scotland (Scottish Council for Voluntary Organisations, SCVO) and Northern Ireland (Northern Ireland Council for Voluntary Action, NICVA).

NCVO provides information and advice to voluntary organisations, through its HelpDesk, publications, magazine, events, and information networks.

NCVO
Regent's Wharf
8 All Saint's Street
London
N1 9RL
Tel: 0207 713 6161
Fax: 0207 713 6300
Website: www.ncvo-vol.org.uk

SCVO
18–19 Claremont Crescent
Edinburgh
EH7 4QD
Tel: 0131 556 3882
Fax: 0131 556 0279

WCVA
Baltic House
Mount Stuart Square
Cardiff Bay
CF10 5FH
Tel: 029 2043 1700
Fax: 029 2043 1701

NICVA
127 Ormeau Road
Belfast
BT7 1SH
Tel: 028 9032 1224
Fax: 028 9043 8350

Voluntary Sector National Training Organisation (VSNTO)

The VSNTO provides materials and resources on training. It has also produced a guide (available via its website) *Leading Managers: a guide to management development in the voluntary sector*. This includes a checklist of essential management skills.

Website: www.vsnto.org.uk
or (contact through the relevant National Council for Voluntary Action)